CANCER SURVIVORSHIP:

What I Wish I'd Known Earlier

JESSIE GRUMAN

Cancer Survivorship: What I Wish I'd Known Earlier

For more information: Health Behavior Media, Center for Advancing Health, 2000 Florida Avenue NW, Suite 210, Washington, DC 20009

Published by Health Behavior Media. Health Behavior Media books are published by the Center for Advancing Health.

Visit CFAH's website at www.cfah.org.

ISBN: 978-0-9815794-4-3

This collection is dedicated to the hundreds of people who have been treated for cancer whose experiences are reflected here. It is a real challenge, in the years following a cancer diagnosis, to assemble an approach to health that protects us from the lingering effects of both the disease and the treatment and alerts us to a recurrence or new cancer. While we all need some basic monitoring, our histories and preferences suggest that survivorship care should be customized to meet our unique needs. Unfortunately, despite investment in developing that field, we find ourselves seeing clinicians who do not recognize the many dimensions of survivorship care, who don't feel qualified to provide it or who are simply not interested in doing so.

I am grateful to those who recounted their stories of survivorship care with me. Each one was a generous reporter, articulate about the strengths and shortcomings of their clinicians and the delivery of their care, but no less eloquent about his or her own culpability in not seeking out or sticking with their post-treatment cancer care plans.

I am honored by their trust in me, which allows me to share their stories with you.

Table of Contents

Introduction

I have been treated for five different cancer diagnoses. Some would call me a cancer survivor.

I call me lucky.

The term "survivor" began to be applied to people who had been treated for cancer in the early '80s in an attempt to capture the unique effects of diagnosis and treatment and the consequent psychological, social and health care needs. As more of us live long lives following treatment and as evidence is gathered about the recurrence of cancer and late effects of treatment, this word now denotes — in the minds of some — very specific phenomena and needs.

However, most people don't know that survivor is medical jargon, rich in meaning for professionals. The public and the media use the word casually, often attaching (or inferring) attributions like "heroic" and "courageous" to describe anyone who has ever received a cancer diagnosis.

That bogus credit leads me and many others who have been treated for cancer to become a little tetchy about being called a cancer survivor.

But as a person who is lucky so far, I know that an accepted, shared term — cancer survivorship — is needed to expand what are now legitimate academic and clinical fields of inquiry and care for those who have been treated for cancer. Knowledge about the long-term effects of cancer and its treatments is advancing steadily. Systematic observations mount about the effects of cancer and its treatment in our bodies and minds as we age, acquire new diseases and undergo the stresses of, oh, life. As more of us live long after our treatment ends, the predictability of our needs for monitoring different organ systems is becoming firmer. We are at increased risk for disease and some of us experience enduring symptoms and effects of treatment for years.

Advances in knowledge about the impact of cancer diagnosis and treatment also signal that each of us should buck up and take on some additional health-related responsibilities over our lifetimes that most of us would prefer to ignore.

This was a surprise to me. For the longest time, I believed that the Hodgkin's lymphoma that was diagnosed on my 20th birthday was a one-off, one-shot deal that had been cured by aggressive treatment, never to be heard from again. Two subsequent cancers discovered early through routine screening were treated surgically. In between these diagnoses in 1992 and 2001, I was robustly healthy. My two most recent diagnoses — gastric and lung cancers — are almost certainly related to the treatment I received for my first cancer diagnosis.

I used to be convinced that survivorship was something that I could attend to for the first couple of years following treatment, after which I could drift off into believing that life and health would proceed as though cancer had never happened.

When I finished my treatment for Hodgkin's lymphoma, the notion of cancer "survivorship" had yet to be coined. My doctor told me to go out and have a good life, come see him if I was ever back in town and reassured me that I would be the first to know if something was wrong. I wanted to believe him, and I did for a while. But eventually I realized I had to be a little more active on my own behalf. While for a long time I was pretty clumsy about how I cared for myself, I have learned a lot the hard way about what it takes to put together a survivorship plan that gives me the best chance to live well with the increasing burden of new cancers and the late effects of previous treatments. As part of my work, I have listened to scores of people who have been treated for cancer and compared notes on our approaches to our experiences with and following cancer treatment.

In these essays, I reflect on *what I wish I'd known earlier about getting good care following active cancer treatment*, based on my own experience and what I have learned from others. There are excellent resources now available to help anyone diagnosed with cancer find their way toward a good survivorship plan. I will reference these when relevant, but, you know, those websites and books and pamphlets are only tools. For those tools to be effective, each of us has to pick them up and use them for our own benefit.

I Wish I'd Known Earlier...

How Fear Can Get in the Way of Cancer Survivorship Care

A recent *Wall Street Journal* article about how post-traumatic stress syndrome can be caused by cancer and stroke brought to mind the variety of responses many people experience after cancer diagnosis and treatment.[1] The lingering intensity of those responses — physical, psychological, social and behavioral — can affect whether and how we attend to the tasks of survivorship; that is, monitoring and addressing the unique health challenges that follow treatment for cancer.

Sam, a friend of mine, told me that his anxiety is starting to rev up about his annual scan to check for a recurrence of his esophageal cancer. It's early July. His appointment is in mid-September. He doesn't want to go. He will force himself to go. He will worry more each day as the test date approaches.

The sound technician for a recent talk I gave recounted how, 17 years after his radical prostatectomy, he insists on having his PSA tested every six months, despite the one-year interval recommended by the guideline. "From the time the blood is drawn to when I get the results I'm still a wreck. And in between tests, my worry is like a pebble in my shoe. It's small, but it's always there."

Some of us are able to approach our survivorship care as just necessary chores. Others have had enough of the cancer experience by the time we have finished treatment: We refuse to participate in any monitoring or testing at all. Some of us — like Sam — muscle through, constantly surfing the waves of worry.

And some of us take matters into our own hands. Like the sound technician, we insist on surgery or medication or we demand more frequent testing than is recommended. We devise our own dietary, physical and mental regimens and employ a range of alternative medicine approaches — sometimes substituting them for standard medical approaches — in an effort to reduce our apprehension and to reclaim some sense that we can control our future.[2,3]

I wish I'd known earlier that a strong emotional response to cancer treatment is fairly common. I recall becoming nauseous at the prospect of walking into a hospital (any hospital!) and the build-up of crushing fear in the days before getting a simple pap test. At first these responses kept me far away from any follow-up care. Then, when my fear of a recurrence exceeded my fear of *testing* for a recurrence, I found myself panicking prior to every check-up, every test. I believed these were rational responses to the highly toxic, aggressive treatment and callous care of an adolescent surprised by a diagnosis of Hodgkin's lymphoma and the threat of impending death at age 20.

Talking with others who experience similar anxieties might have made it seem more normal. A behavioral intervention by a mental health professional could have drained some of the anxiety.

As control of pain and nausea become more effective, perhaps fewer of us will experience such responses. But the diagnosis and treatment of cancer affects each of us differently. Increased recognition by our clinicians of their potential impact, and help finding effective approaches to accommodating our new reality, can calm the waves of emotion that get in the way of returning to the lives we love.

Cancer treatment can affect physical, emotional, cognitive, social, behavioral and occupational aspects of our lives. Survivorship care by definition is care of the whole person.[4]

It sometimes takes my breath away that my own fear could easily have stood in the way of the discovery and treatment of my four subsequent cancers.

I wish I'd known earlier how easy it would be to undermine the possibility of benefitting fully both from the treatment I received and ongoing monitoring and testing because I couldn't see that I needed help with my fear.

I Wish I'd Known Earlier...

Not Every Oncologist Can or Should Deliver Survivorship Care

The first oncologist to provide me with survivorship care would feel the lymph nodes in my neck, ask me how I was feeling ("Fine") and then hold forth for a half-hour about the wrong-headedness of federal research priorities, knowing that I worked at the National Institutes of Health.

Another oncologist I asked to provide me with comprehensive survivorship care balked when I asked him to feel the lymph nodes in my neck. He was an oncological gynecologist and my neck was "not [his] body part." Comprehensive? Ahem.

Another oncologist to whom I was referred for survivorship care took one look at me when I showed up for a routine visit and exclaimed, "What are *you* doing here? I have sick people to take care of! Don't worry, I won't charge you for this visit."

I encountered that first doctor early in the development of cancer survivorship as a focus for oncologists and primary care providers. The second and third were oncologists in major comprehensive cancer centers and were in charge of my survivorship care for extended periods in the late 1990s/early 2000s.

What's up with that? Why was I so willing to be cared for by clinicians who were so poorly matched to the challenges of guiding me as my care grew increasingly complex with each new cancer diagnosis? And why was it so hard to find someone who was actually willing to help me meet those challenges? It's not as though I didn't have a clue what I needed, and it's not as though survivorship care remained an unknown, unimportant part of the job of most oncologists and many primary care clinicians.

We are not the only ones who must be convinced that we have unique health concerns following the active treatment of our cancer. Clinicians must also believe that special care for us is important, and they have to learn how to provide that care. Then they have to take the time to listen to us and help us get the tests we need, find solutions for the sometimes intractable lingering physical, psychological and social symptoms of the disease and treatment, and keep a sharp eye out for late effects and recurrences. This is no small order, especially when time is short and insurance reimbursement can be tricky.

Here's one source of the problem: Recent surveys published in the *Journal of General Internal Medicine* asked primary care clinicians and oncologists who should care for cancer patients once they finish active treatment.[1] Almost two-thirds of oncologists had little confidence in the skills of primary care clinicians to order appropriate tests and treat the late effects of breast cancer treatment. And many primary care clinicians agreed with the oncologists: Only 40 percent of primary care clinicians expressed confidence in their own knowledge about testing for recurrence and late effects. Further, in the survey cited above, although oncologists said that they provided treatment summaries or care plans to primary care clinicians a majority of the time, primary care clinicians reported receiving them a minority of the time.

And so who is it, again, who will take responsibility for our survivorship care?

It would be wonderful if each of our oncologists sat down with us to complete a comprehensive survivorship care plan at the end of our active treatment. It would be even better that they tell us candidly if they are unwilling or unable to work with us to fulfill that plan. If they are either, helping us find someone who is and then formally making the hand-off to them would make a big difference.

In spite of a heavy investment of effort by patient advocacy, professional and government groups with a stake in survivorship care, I don't see this happening soon, especially with the reorganization of health care currently taking place and the workforce constraints mentioned above.[2-5]

This means that for many, a substantial part of the burden of finding good survivorship care may rest with us and our family caregivers. If you are in this situation, take a look at the survivorship guidelines for patients from the National Comprehensive Cancer Network (or the Children's Oncology Group for survivors of pediatric cancers) to see the full breadth and depth of what comprehensive survivorship care looks like.[6,7] You need a template to make sure you and your new doctor are on the same wavelength: Good survivorship care is not just periodic testing and the ritual palpation of lymph nodes.

If asking for a referral where you were treated hasn't worked or you are unsatisfied with your current survivorship care, take a careful trip through the LiveStrong website where you will find good guidance about where to look for it.[8] Similarly, cancer centers supported by the National Cancer Institute — large and small (or the Children's Oncology Group's Late Effects Directory for pediatric survivors) — have survivorship programs that might offer you a choice of physicians who will provide comprehensive survivorship care.[9-11]

Curiously, none of my subsequent cancers were detected by examining my lymph nodes. Some have been found via routine screenings based on survivorship guidelines, the others only through the vigilance of a unique physician who specializes in follow-up care for those treated for pediatric cancers.

It's a sad surprise to realize that even if you can overcome your fear of recurrence or general resistance to more cancer-related health care, getting yourself the survivorship care that researchers and experts agree you need may not be that easy.[12]

I wish I'd known earlier that I was going to need to work at getting good survivorship care. And even more, I wish I didn't have to.

I Wish I'd Known Earlier...

For Many of Us, Symptoms and Late Effects Accumulate Rather Than Fade Over Time

Sara was treated for multiple myeloma in the mid-90s and had a stem cell transplant seven years ago. When I asked her husband how she was doing, he said, "Pretty well... just the gift of a little edema in one arm and some neuropathy in her feet."

On one hand you think, "Hey! That's great! Those little gifts — those side effects — are a small price to pay." On the other hand, seven years of edema and neuropathy for an active hiking enthusiast are nothing to sneeze at.

The side effects of cancer treatment sometimes fade but can become permanent glitches — disturbing symptoms whose impact we try to mitigate and whose presence we attempt to accommodate.

If you know someone who was treated for cancer in the 1970s or 1980s, you might be aware of the effects of early, very aggressive treatments that have emerged over time: the stooped shoulders, weak neck muscles, heart ailments, swallowing difficulties and secondary cancers that accrue to what is now known to be excessive radiation treatment. You can also imagine that the long-term risks of many of today's newest cancer treatments are as yet unknown.

As evidence builds from the long-term follow-up of people treated in clinical trials in the latter part of the last century, knowledge about the risks of those outmoded treatments has become more systematized. "Oh, this is classic in Hodgkin's patients treated in those days," remarked a rehabilitation physician when examining my weakening back muscles. "We see it starting anywhere after 20 years post-radiation treatment."

You know the evidence is gathering about your disease treatment when its late effect profile includes the term "classic." You also begin to hope that new, more effective and less risky treatment approaches are being developed.

For a long time, I believed that cancer and the effects of its treatment were containable, that the tincture of time would minimize their impact on the length and quality of my life. I thought that survivorship care consisted of regular testing to see whether I had a recurrence or a new primary cancer. My imagination accorded little space for the compromises in physical, cognitive or social functioning that become more pronounced over time or that burst into existence as I age due to either my cancer diagnoses or their treatments.

I don't wish that I'd known about the full, exciting range of diseases, disorders and disabilities for which I am now at risk. It wouldn't have mattered anyway: Denial is my favorite defense and I no doubt would have deployed it efficiently.

I do wish, however, that I had had a more fulsome orientation to the trajectory and value of survivorship care. I think it would have been helpful to understand that the symptoms and late effects for many cancer patients often accumulate over time, rather than fade to nothing. It is not only the fact that I have had cancer but the particulars of my treatment that increase my risks. If I understood this, I would have placed greater value in working with clinicians who view new symptoms and conditions through the lens of cancer survivorship, rather than independently occurring phenomenon.

Of course, not every person who has been treated for cancer would find this orientation worthwhile. Many people are treated for early-stage cancers — some of which may soon not even be identified as cancer — and they will live out my naive idea of how this should work... the tincture of time, the fading of the effects of surgery and minimal chemotherapy or radiation.[1] For them, survivorship care is a matter of vigilance for five years post-treatment before fading back into the risk profile of the normal population.

For the rest of us, from childhood survivors on up, settling into the notion that cancer diagnosis and treatment are "gifts that keep on giving" requires a long-term commitment by both the individual and the survivorship clinician to identify the next manifestation of that gift and to seek innovative approaches to ensuring that it detracts as little as possible from the quality and length of our lives.

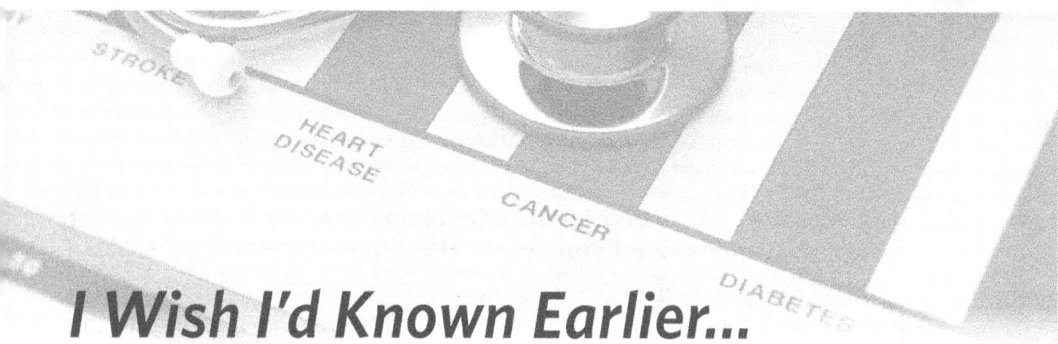

I Wish I'd Known Earlier...

To Cast a Cool Eye on Prognostic and Risk Statistics

> I made the decision to try nonmedical approaches to healing my
> early breast cancer for quite a while. It was not what my doctor
> recommended, but there was a much bigger chance that it would
> not metastasize than it would, and I took a risk that I would be one
> of the lucky ones. Eventually I had to have a mastectomy. — Kate,
> 39, personal trainer

For many of us, receiving a cancer diagnosis includes hearing statistics
about the average or median survival of people with this stage of this
type of cancer. The end of active treatment may arrive accompanied by
additional statistics: the risk of recurrence, of different late effects, of
secondary cancers.

It is difficult, even for those schooled in the meaning of such numbers,
to figure out what they mean for an individual. Some choose not to even
try. And not figuring it out can lead, as demonstrated above, not only to
miscalculations and odd choices but also to a surge in anxiety.

Stephen Jay Gould, evolutionary scientist and prolific author, wrote
about his own encounter with survival statistics when diagnosed with
abdominal mesothelioma, a rare and serious cancer usually associated
with exposure to asbestos. When his doctor told him there wasn't much
about it to be found in the medical literature, Gould did his own search,
only to find that the median survival for this disease was eight months.
He panicked.

Then Gould fell back on his statistical training: That median mortality
didn't mean that he would be dead in eight months, but rather that
half of people known to have the disease die within eight months of its

diagnosis. Further, an equal number of people lived for eight months or longer, and Gould shared a number of characteristics of those who lived longer: He was young and strong. And finally, the survival statistic was based on people who received conventional modes of treatment, and Gould was being treated with the latest experimental protocol. He was convinced that the eight-month prognosis didn't apply to him and that he "would have time to think, to plan, to fight."

Gould died at age 60, 20 years following this diagnosis — from a different type of cancer.

I am not Stephen Jay Gould. I have neither the breadth of knowledge nor the training to sort through the statistics I am given or that I seek out in order to get a clearer picture of what a diagnosis might truly mean for me. I know that I am prone to panic when I hear survival statistics about my new diagnosis. And once heard, I cannot un-hear them, even though I can do my damndest to convince myself that they are not relevant to me, as they were not to Gould.

In truth, this is not simple even for my physicians: The translation of ratios that represent the experience of groups into the implications for an individual is always difficult. What factors should be taken into account when you customize such statistics for an individual? How much valence does each have?

I wish I'd known earlier to view survival statistics particularly and risk statistics generally at a cool remove. I have had to learn to see them as a sign to be vigilant but not a personalized prediction about the length and quality of my life. I have had to let go of my need to think I could gain some control of future days by ferreting out this kind of information: So far, it has offered only false promises and unnecessary heartbreak.

I have had to learn to step away from the statistics and focus on the day — sometimes the hour — in front of me.

I Wish I'd Known Earlier...

I Still Need a Primary Care Provider Since Most Headaches Aren't Brain Tumors

Having cancer has infected me and many others with the irritating tendency to view any persistent, troubling symptom through the lens of a recurrence or a diagnosis of a new primary cancer. A friend of mine who is nearly five years post-kidney cancer treatment casually remarked the other day that he needed to see a doctor about his sore ankle: It could be arthritis, but it might be cancer, of course. Someone I interviewed recently commented that despite the ten years since her treatment for breast cancer, she frequently has to convince herself that each new symptom that crops up is not evidence of another catastrophic cancer diagnosis.

Many people lose track of their primary care clinicians when they are deep into their cancer treatment. Indeed, it's probably the case that with the exception of chronic conditions like diabetes and heart disease, many of the health disturbances we experience during this time are treatment-related and are best handled by our oncologist or through a direct referral — often to a specialist, interestingly. But in the midst of an episode of cancer treatment, it sure is more convenient to get a prescription for a urinary tract infection from a clinician to whom you are talking all the time and who has your up-to-date information.

I wish I'd known earlier that once active treatment is over, that if I'm getting my survivorship care from my treating oncologist or other survivorship specialist, I have to find myself a primary care clinician who knows my health history. Why? Because despite the wallop packed by cancer treatment, I still am vulnerable to all the germs and stresses and injuries to which everyone else of my age and sex is subject. My primary care clinician needs to be someone who is familiar with complicated patients like me, not someone who will regard me as a new exotic specimen. Only then will she be able to separate for herself and for me whatever symptoms I have from a recurrence of my cancer (or a new one). Only then will I be able to benefit from the broad array of approaches and tools of primary care.

I have at times, out of sheer inertia, fear or laziness, tried to use my various oncologists to deliver rudimentary primary care. This has proved to be a bad idea. It's difficult to get in to see them anyway and once you are there, they tend to say things like "I don't know anything about the flu," or "Don't you have a primary care doctor? You should get one." And lately, as I have been the recipient of good primary care, I have come to see the risks I took by not having my health care coordinated by a general practitioner.

This tendency for even minor symptoms to set off a mild (or major) panic is not trivial for many of us. I am particularly prone to this kind of thinking these days because my two most recent cancer diagnoses came after my attempts to treat minor symptoms as such were cut short by my vigilant survivorship doctor and they turned out to be gastric and lung cancer respectively.

But such thinking can lead us to hang on to our oncologist-anchors at a time when a good connection with a primary care clinician has the potential to prevent, manage and treat other conditions (flu! pneumonia! accidents!). Such a connection can help us regain our perspective and confidence about our health so we can sustain our efforts to live interesting, active lives.

I Wish I'd Known Earlier...

Survivorship Care Is a Mutual Enterprise

I wish I'd known earlier that survivorship care is neither a do-it-yourself project nor is it something that I can simply hand off to experts. There is no stable set of signs, signals and test protocols that, if followed assiduously — and that come up negative — means I am protected from a recurrence, new cancer or late effects of treatment. Observation, expertise and self-knowledge from both me and my doctor are critical to getting the best follow-up care.

As former cancer patients, we can't just walk in to our appointments with our oncologist, survivorship specialist or primary care doctor every six months or year and have survivorship care handled for us. Far from it. We are the historians of our health. Only we can observe the fluctuations in our functioning and report on the symptoms that underlie them. Only we can describe our reactions to drugs and procedures. Only we can verify the accuracy of our records. Only we can actually show up, follow through on testing and experiment with fixes to see what might work for us.

But the context in which we take those actions becomes more complicated with each passing year. Treatment trials find new patterns of risk for late effects, and new approaches to treating late effects are developed. Some of this takes place within oncology, but much of it takes place in related disciplines: cardiology, endocrinology, rehabilitation medicine, physical therapy. Keeping a critical finger on the pulse of those developments is a nice hobby for those patients with the time and interest, but the responsibility for really knowing what's going on in those fields belongs to my survivorship doctor or care team rather than to me.

This is a mutual enterprise, my survivorship care. Without me, my careful monitoring of my own health and willingness to act to find good solutions, my doctor has nothing to work with. Without my doctor, his careful monitoring of research developments, his wealth of experience with other patients and his ability to personalize what he knows for my unique history, I have no guidance to discover and address the long-term effects of cancer treatment.

If you are a cancer survivor, you know how the panic of a new diagnosis sparks a promise to do whatever it takes to return to health and then to take really good care of yourself so this never happens again.

Right?

A few years after I finished treatment for my first diagnosis, Hodgkin's lymphoma, I finally came around to thinking that getting someone to provide survivorship care was probably a good idea, but I was having trouble finding someone to provide it.[1] "Well OK," I thought, "I'll just have to do this myself." And so I gave it a whirl. In a fit of industriousness, I searched for journal articles about long-term results from relevant treatment trials and tracked down treatment guidelines. I talked to oncologists and staff at the National Cancer Institute and the American Cancer Society and put together a list of tests to get and symptoms to look out for. Then I got distracted by, oh, life and attended to my plan when I remembered to...when I had time. And because I had this little plan in place, my enthusiasm for finding a physician who would deliver real survivorship care ebbed.

This would be a better story if I could tell you that I paid dearly for my casual approach to my care. But I didn't. I lucked out and had an uneventful healthy few years. However, when I finally found a good survivorship doctor, he spent two full hours going over just what I was at risk for and what I could do about it. I felt chills go down my spine.

How could I have missed all that information? How could I have overlooked whole organ systems and recommendations for monitoring and testing? Minor health disturbances (heart problems, swallowing, neck weakness), when seen through the lens of survivorship, had explanations and solutions, whereas before they were random signs of aging. How could I have forgotten those promises I made to myself about really taking good care of my health each time I'd been diagnosed with a new primary cancer? How could I have put myself at such risk?

We all make promises to ourselves we can't keep (think New Year's resolutions) and the ones we make while terrified by a new cancer diagnosis are probably no more or less likely to stick. But the one many of us make to take better care of ourselves needs to include our active participation in our survivorship care. We must find a good survivorship care clinician/team that can join us in our effort to live for as long and as well as we can.

I Wish I'd Known Earlier...

Each New Diagnosis Has Unique Demands

Ever heard the saying "You never step into the same river twice"?

It has taken me a long time to apply its meaning to my experiences with five different forms of cancer as well as a variety of serious late effects of my treatments.

Each time I get the news of a new diagnosis, I have tended to fall into the trap of thinking that since I know a lot about the kinds of cancer I have had, and even more about being a cancer patient, I can predict exactly what this next adventure will be like. Given the amount practice I've had, that reaction is understandable.

But it is also dangerous. I can (and do) scare myself silly or confront my situation with far-too-casual equanimity, depending on which memories I dredge up. Some of the memories are pleasant (the relief of finishing treatment, the camaraderie in the radiology waiting room) while others remain horrifying (a painful surgery, a bad drug reaction). Because cancer treatment at its best is inconvenient and at its worst is uncomfortable and disabling, the bad memories tend to crowd out the good.

But neither a casual nor a frightened response is particularly useful when, once again, I am thrown into that post-diagnostic uncertainty. I can't afford to rush into hasty, unconsidered actions based on one test or one doctor's recommendation, and I can't afford to minimize the threat and head off for a month's vacation before I put a plan together.

During such times, I wish I could remember that while a familiar river may look the same each time I gaze at it, the water flowing between its banks is not. While on the surface, the disease or symptom may appear to be similar to past diagnoses, it is not the same. It is different first of all because each new symptom, late effect or cancer diagnosis is taking place in a body that has been scanned and drugged and radiated and surgically rearranged. Cancer changes us; its treatment changes us; other non-cancer disease processes change us. Time changes us. So each new diagnosis, symptom or problem places unique demands on us.

It's also different because the diagnosis and treatment of cancer and associated late effects are changing all the time. I may think I know how the monitoring of thyroid irregularities is approached based on my experience six years ago but I find out I'm wrong. I may think I really understand how to take anti-emetics post-chemotherapy but the cocktail of drugs and their timing is different now, not only because the general approach in the scientific literature has changed but because I have a new doctor and a new kind of cancer and a new chemotherapy regimen.

And it's different because I am different. Time has passed since my last diagnosis. I have once again absorbed and accommodated the limitations cancer has imposed.

And so, even as practiced as I am, I've found that actually finding the right care and then making the most of that care has to be discovered *de novo* each time a new condition or symptom is revealed.

Yes, there is much that I have learned that remains the same: I know I need to resist making decisions without careful consideration of alternatives; that I must educate myself about my condition and treatment options; that I should share the news with others about my health selectively and carefully; that the chaos I feel following a bad diagnosis will eventually reside and I will return to some semblance of the life I love; that I must ask for help.

I am deeply familiar with the *process* I must go through when I receive a new diagnosis, but I wish I had known earlier that knowing about the process provides no shortcut for the sheer hard work that we patients must do to fill in the details — the *content* — that will bring us to and through good treatment. Rather, what I can be sure of is that I am not an expert in what is to come and that the new diagnosis is a signal to gather my energy and say to myself, "Hey! I need to know about all the new water flowing through that old riverbed."

References

I Wish I'd Known Earlier... How Fear Can Get in the Way of Cancer Survivorship Care

1. When Disease Can Bring on PTSD. Wall Street Journal. June 24, 2013. http://online.wsj.com/article/SB10001424127887323998604578565 580703412550.html

2. Diet May Cut Risk of Cancer Recurring. Washington Post. May 17, 2005. http://www.washingtonpost.com/wp-dyn/content/ article/2005/05/16/AR2005051600353.html

3. Meditation and Cancer Patients. WABC New York. March 21, 2011. http://abclocal.go.com/wabc/story?section=news/ health&id=8025122

4. Cancer Care for the Whole Patient: Meeting Psychosocial Health Needs. Institute of Medicine. October 15, 2007. http://www.iom.edu/Reports/2007/Cancer-Care-for-the-Whole-Patient-Meeting-Psychosocial-Health-Needs.aspx

I Wish I'd Known Earlier... Not Every Oncologist Can or Should Deliver Survivorship Care

1. Differences Between Primary Care Physicians' and Oncologists' Knowledge, Attitudes and Practices Regarding the Care of Cancer Survivors. Journal of General Internal Medicine. December 2011. http://link.springer.com/article/10.1007%2Fs11606-011-1808-4

2. National Coalition for Cancer Survivorship. http://www.canceradvocacy.org/

3. CancerCare. http://www.cancercare.org/

4. American Society of Clinical Oncology. http://www.asco.org/

5. Office of Cancer Survivorship, National Cancer Institute. http://cancercontrol.cancer.gov/ocs/

6. National Comprehensive Cancer Network. http://www.nccn.org/professionals/physician_gls/f_guidelines. asp#survivorship

7. Children's Oncology Group. http://www.survivorshipguidelines.org/

8. LiveStrong Survivorship Centers of Excellence. http://www.livestrong.org/What-We-Do/Our-Actions/Programs-Partnerships/LIVESTRONG-Survivorship-Centers-of-Excellence

9. Find a Cancer Center. National Cancer Institute. http://www.cancer.gov/researchandfunding/extramural/cancercenters/find-a-cancer-center

10. NCI Community Cancer Centers Program: 2012 NCCCP Hospitals http://ncccp.cancer.gov/about/sites.htm

11. Late Effects Directory of Services. Children's Oncology Group. http://applications.childrensoncologygroup.org/Surveys/lateEffects/lateEffects.PublicSearch.asp

12. I Wish I'd Known Earlier... How Fear Can Get in the Way of Cancer Survivorship Care. Center for Advancing Health. July 17, 2013. http://www.cfah.org/blog/2013/i-wish-i-had-known-earlierhow-fear-can-get-in-the-way-of-cancer-survivorship-care

I Wish I'd Known Earlier... For Many of Us, Symptoms and Late Effects Accumulate Rather Than Fade Over Time

1. Experts Call for Redefinition of 'Cancer'. HealthDay. July 30, 2013. http://consumer.healthday.com/cancer-information-5/mis-cancer-news-102/experts-advise-redefinition-of-cancer-678739.html

I Wish I'd Known Earlier... Survivorship Care Is a Mutual Enterprise

1. I Wish I'd Known Earlier... Not Every Oncologist Can or Should Deliver Survivorship Care. Center for Advancing Health. July 24, 2013. http://www.cfah.org/blog/2013/i-wish-i-had-known-earlier-not-every-oncologist-can-or-should-deliver-survivorship-care

Jessie Gruman

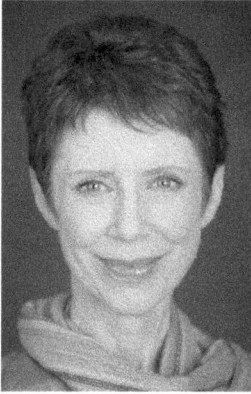

Jessie Gruman is president and founder of the Center for Advancing Health, a nonpartisan, Washington-based policy institute which, since 1992, has been supported by foundations and individuals to work on people's engagement in their health care from the patient perspective. Dr. Gruman draws on her own experience of treatment for five cancer diagnoses, interviews with patients and caregivers, surveys and peer-reviewed research as the basis of her work to describe and advocate for policies and practices to overcome the challenges people face in finding good care and getting the most from it.

Gruman has worked on this same set of concerns in the private sector (AT&T), the public sector (National Cancer Institute) and the voluntary health sector (American Cancer Society).

She is a member of the American Academy of Arts and Sciences and the Council on Foreign Relations and is a fellow of the New York Academy of Medicine and the Society for Behavioral Medicine. She was honored by Research!America for her leadership in advocacy for health research and has received honorary doctorates from Brown University, Carnegie Mellon University, Clark University, Georgetown University, New York University, Northeastern University, Salve Regina University, Syracuse University and Tulane University, and the Presidential Medal of the George Washington University.

Gruman holds a B.A. from Vassar College and a Ph.D. in Social Psychology from Columbia University and is a Professorial Lecturer in the School of Public Health and Health Services at the George Washington University.

Dr. Gruman is the author of *AfterShock: What to Do When the Doctor Gives You – or Someone You Love – a Devastating Diagnosis* (Walker Publishing, second edition, 2010); *Slow Leaks: Missed Opportunities to Encourage Our Engagement in Our Health Care* (Health Behavior Media, 2013); *A Year of Living Sickishly: A Patient Reflects* (Health Behavior Media, 2013); *The Experience of the American Patient: Risk, Trust and Choice* (Health Behavior Media, 2009); *Behavior Matters* (Health Behavior Media, 2008) as well as scientific papers and opinion essays and articles. She blogs regularly on the Prepared Patient Blog and tweets daily @jessiegruman.